This Book Belongs to

_____

_____

START / END DATES

/ / _____ TO / / _____

To see more books from Louise Curtis
SCAN HERE

"Ability is what you're capable of doing.
Motivation determines what you do.
Attitude determines how well you do it."

Lou Holtz

What is Intermittent fasting?

Intermittent Fasting is a popular way of losing weight by restricting food intake for a pre-determined period of time, thus reducing your calorie intake.

There are several methods of fasting.

- The 16:8 Method: This is the most popular method. You fast for 16 hours and then you are permitted to eat for 8 hours. Usually, this method is to fast overnight until lunchtime. Eat a healthy lunch and dinner, taking note of the time you finish eating then fast until 16 hours have passed. Only water, black tea, and coffee are taken during this fasting time.
- The 5:2 Method: You eat normally for 5 days of the week, then restrict your intake to about 500 calories for 2 days a week.
- The Eat Stop Eat Method: This was popularized by fitness expert Brad Pilon. Choose one or two non-consecutive 24 hour periods to fast by not eating at all on those days.
- Alternate Day Fasting: This method involves fasting about every other day by restricting your calories to 0 or 500 calories. This is not a popular method as studies have shown that it is no more effective than a normal calorie-restrictive diet.
- The Warrior Diet: This method involves eating only small amounts of fruits and vegetables during the day and then eating a big meal at night.
- OMAD: One Meal A Day. This is a popular way of fasting because you only eat for 1 hour per day. This can be very effective especially if you combine your fasting with eating Low Carb foods, cutting out sugars, flour, and starchy vegetables.

For most of these programs you would choose your fast hours or days to suit your own schedule and lifestyle.

"You didn't gain all your weight in one day; you won't lose it in one day. Be patient with yourself."

Jenna Wolfe

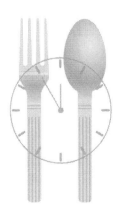

Weight and Measurement Tracker

DATE	Upper Arm	Chest	Thigh	Abdomen	Hips	Weight	+/-

Weight and Measurement Tracker

DATE	Upper Arm	Chest	Thigh	Abdomen	Hips	Weight	+/-

Weight and Measurement Tracker

DATE	Upper Arm	Chest	Thigh	Abdomen	Hips	Weight	+/-

Weight and Measurement Tracker

DATE	Upper Arm	Chest	Thigh	Abdomen	Hips	Weight	+/-

Monthly Fasting Tracker

DATE	EATING FROM	EATING TO	TOTAL HOURS	FASTING FROM	FASTING TO	FASTING HOURS	DONE

Monthly Fasting Tracker

DATE	EATING FROM	EATING TO	TOTAL HOURS	FASTING FROM	FASTING TO	FASTING HOURS	DONE

Monthly Fasting Tracker

"Wisdom is doing now what you are going to be happy with later on." - Joyce Meyer

DATE	EATING FROM	EATING TO	TOTAL HOURS	FASTING FROM	FASTING TO	FASTING HOURS	DONE

Monthly Fasting Tracker

DATE	EATING FROM	EATING TO	TOTAL HOURS	FASTING FROM	FASTING TO	FASTING HOURS	DONE

Intermittent Fasting Tracker

DAY		DATE		FASTING DAY	Y N	WEIGHT	

FIRST BITE		FASTING HOURS	
LAST BITE		EATING HOURS	

SLEEP

TO BED		HOURS	
WOKE UP		SLEPT	

EXERCISE QUALITY

TIME		TYPE		DURATION	

MEAL / SNACK	TIME	CALORIES
	TOTAL	

ENERGY LEVEL

☆☆☆☆☆
☆☆☆☆☆

WATER INTAKE (GLASSES)

⬭⬭⬭⬭
⬭⬭⬭⬭

NOTES

"If it is important to you, you will find a way. If not, you'll find an excuse."
-Unknown

Intermittent Fasting Tracker

DAY		DATE		FASTING DAY	Y N	WEIGHT	

FIRST BITE			FASTING HOURS	
LAST BITE			EATING HOURS	

SLEEP				
TO BED			HOURS	
WOKE UP			SLEPT	

EXERCISE			QUALITY	
TIME		TYPE		DURATION

MEAL / SNACK	TIME	CALORIES
		TOTAL

ENERGY LEVEL	NOTES
☆☆☆☆☆	
☆☆☆☆☆	

WATER INTAKE (GLASSES)

◊ ◊ ◊ ◊
◊ ◊ ◊ ◊

"It does not matter how slowly you go as long as you do not stop."
-Confucious

Intermittent Fasting Tracker

DAY		DATE		FASTING DAY	Y N	WEIGHT

FIRST BITE		FASTING HOURS	
LAST BITE		EATING HOURS	

SLEEP

TO BED		HOURS	
WOKE UP		SLEPT	

EXERCISE QUALITY

TIME		TYPE		DURATION	

MEAL / SNACK	TIME	CALORIES
	TOTAL	

ENERGY LEVEL

☆☆☆☆☆
☆☆☆☆☆

WATER INTAKE (GLASSES)

◇◇◇◇
◇◇◇◇

NOTES

"If it is important to you,
you will find a way. If
not, you'll find an excuse."
-Unknown

Intermittent Fasting Tracker

DAY		DATE		FASTING DAY	Y N	WEIGHT	

FIRST BITE		FASTING HOURS	
LAST BITE		EATING HOURS	

SLEEP

TO BED		HOURS	
WOKE UP		SLEPT	

EXERCISE QUALITY

TIME		TYPE		DURATION	

MEAL / SNACK	TIME	CALORIES
	TOTAL	

ENERGY LEVEL

☆☆☆☆☆
☆☆☆☆☆

WATER INTAKE (GLASSES)

◊◊◊◊
◊◊◊◊

NOTES

"It does not matter how slowly you go as long as you do not stop."
-Confucious

Intermittent Fasting Tracker

DAY		DATE		FASTING DAY	Y N	WEIGHT

FIRST BITE		FASTING HOURS	
LAST BITE		EATING HOURS	

SLEEP

TO BED		HOURS	
WOKE UP		SLEPT	

EXERCISE		QUALITY	
TIME		TYPE		DURATION	

MEAL / SNACK	TIME	CALORIES
	TOTAL	

ENERGY LEVEL	NOTES
☆☆☆☆☆ ☆☆☆☆☆	

WATER INTAKE (GLASSES)

◊◊◊◊
◊◊◊◊

"If it is important to you, you will find a way. If not, you'll find an excuse."
-Unknown

Intermittent Fasting Tracker

DAY		DATE		FASTING DAY	Y N	WEIGHT	

FIRST BITE			FASTING HOURS	
LAST BITE			EATING HOURS	

SLEEP				
TO BED			HOURS	
WOKE UP			SLEPT	

EXERCISE			QUALITY	
TIME		TYPE		DURATION	

MEAL / SNACK	TIME	CALORIES
	TOTAL	

ENERGY LEVEL

☆☆☆☆☆
☆☆☆☆☆

WATER INTAKE (GLASSES)

◯◯◯◯
◯◯◯◯

NOTES

"It does not matter how slowly you go as long as you do not stop."
-Confucious

Intermittent Fasting Tracker

DAY		DATE		FASTING DAY	Y N	WEIGHT	

FIRST BITE		FASTING HOURS	
LAST BITE		EATING HOURS	

SLEEP

TO BED		HOURS	
WOKE UP		SLEPT	

EXERCISE   QUALITY

TIME		TYPE		DURATION	

MEAL / SNACK	TIME	CALORIES
	TOTAL	

ENERGY LEVEL

☆☆☆☆☆
☆☆☆☆☆

WATER INTAKE (GLASSES)

◯◯◯◯
◯◯◯◯

NOTES

"If it is important to you, you will find a way. If not, you'll find an excuse."
-Unknown

Intermittent Fasting Tracker

DAY		DATE		FASTING DAY	Y N	WEIGHT	
FIRST BITE			FASTING HOURS				
LAST BITE			EATING HOURS				

SLEEP

TO BED		HOURS	
WOKE UP		SLEPT	

EXERCISE		QUALITY			
TIME		TYPE		DURATION	

MEAL / SNACK	TIME	CALORIES
	TOTAL	

ENERGY LEVEL	NOTES
☆☆☆☆☆ ☆☆☆☆☆	

WATER INTAKE (GLASSES)

◊ ◊ ◊ ◊
◊ ◊ ◊ ◊

"It does not matter how slowly you go as long as you do not stop."
-Confucious

Intermittent Fasting Tracker

DAY		DATE		FASTING DAY	Y N	WEIGHT

FIRST BITE		FASTING HOURS	
LAST BITE		EATING HOURS	

SLEEP

TO BED		HOURS	
WOKE UP		SLEPT	

EXERCISE — **QUALITY**

TIME		TYPE		DURATION	

MEAL / SNACK	TIME	CALORIES
	TOTAL	

ENERGY LEVEL	NOTES
☆☆☆☆☆	
☆☆☆☆☆	

WATER INTAKE (GLASSES)

◇ ◇ ◇ ◇
◇ ◇ ◇ ◇

"If it is important to you, you will find a way. If not, you'll find an excuse."
-Unknown

Intermittent Fasting Tracker

DAY		DATE		FASTING DAY	Y N	WEIGHT	
FIRST BITE			FASTING HOURS				
LAST BITE			EATING HOURS				

SLEEP

TO BED		HOURS	
WOKE UP		SLEPT	

EXERCISE | QUALITY

TIME		TYPE		DURATION	

MEAL / SNACK	TIME	CALORIES
	TOTAL	

ENERGY LEVEL

☆☆☆☆☆
☆☆☆☆☆

WATER INTAKE (GLASSES)

◊ ◊ ◊ ◊
◊ ◊ ◊ ◊

NOTES

"It does not matter how slowly you go as long as you do not stop."
-Confucious

Intermittent Fasting Tracker

DAY		DATE		FASTING DAY	Y N	WEIGHT	

FIRST BITE		FASTING HOURS	
LAST BITE		EATING HOURS	

SLEEP

TO BED		HOURS	
WOKE UP		SLEPT	

EXERCISE | | | **QUALITY**

TIME		TYPE		DURATION	

MEAL / SNACK	TIME	CALORIES
		TOTAL

ENERGY LEVEL	NOTES
☆☆☆☆☆ ☆☆☆☆☆	
WATER INTAKE (GLASSES)	
⬡⬡⬡⬡ ⬡⬡⬡⬡	

"If it is important to you, you will find a way. If not, you'll find an excuse."
-Unknown

Intermittent Fasting Tracker

| DAY | | DATE | | FASTING DAY | Y N | WEIGHT | |

| FIRST BITE | | FASTING HOURS | |
| LAST BITE | | EATING HOURS | |

SLEEP

| TO BED | | HOURS | |
| WOKE UP | | SLEPT | |

| EXERCISE | QUALITY |
| TIME | TYPE | DURATION |

MEAL / SNACK	TIME	CALORIES
		TOTAL

ENERGY LEVEL	NOTES
☆☆☆☆☆	
☆☆☆☆☆	

WATER INTAKE (GLASSES)

◊ ◊ ◊ ◊
◊ ◊ ◊ ◊

"It does not matter how slowly you go as long as you do not stop."
-Confucious

Intermittent Fasting Tracker

DAY		DATE		FASTING DAY	Y N	WEIGHT
FIRST BITE			FASTING HOURS			
LAST BITE			EATING HOURS			

SLEEP

TO BED			HOURS	
WOKE UP			SLEPT	

EXERCISE			QUALITY	
TIME		TYPE		DURATION

MEAL / SNACK	TIME	CALORIES
		TOTAL

ENERGY LEVEL

☆☆☆☆☆
☆☆☆☆☆

WATER INTAKE (GLASSES)

⬤⬤⬤⬤
⬤⬤⬤⬤

NOTES

"If it is important to you, you will find a way. If not, you'll find an excuse."
-Unknown

Intermittent Fasting Tracker

DAY		DATE		FASTING DAY	Y N	WEIGHT	

FIRST BITE		FASTING HOURS	
LAST BITE		EATING HOURS	

SLEEP

TO BED		HOURS	
WOKE UP		SLEPT	

EXERCISE		QUALITY	
TIME		TYPE		DURATION	

MEAL / SNACK	TIME	CALORIES
	TOTAL	

ENERGY LEVEL

☆☆☆☆☆
☆☆☆☆☆

WATER INTAKE (GLASSES)

◇◇◇◇
◇◇◇◇

NOTES

"It does not matter how slowly you go as long as you do not stop."
-Confucious

Intermittent Fasting Tracker

DAY		DATE		FASTING DAY	Y N	WEIGHT	

FIRST BITE		FASTING HOURS	
LAST BITE		EATING HOURS	

SLEEP			
TO BED		HOURS	
WOKE UP		SLEPT	

EXERCISE		QUALITY	
TIME		TYPE		DURATION	

MEAL / SNACK	TIME	CALORIES
		TOTAL

ENERGY LEVEL	NOTES
☆☆☆☆☆	
☆☆☆☆☆	

WATER INTAKE (GLASSES)

⬤ ⬤ ⬤ ⬤
⬤ ⬤ ⬤ ⬤

"If it is important to you, you will find a way. If not, you'll find an excuse."
-Unknown

Intermittent Fasting Tracker

DAY		DATE		FASTING DAY	Y N	WEIGHT	

FIRST BITE		FASTING HOURS	
LAST BITE		EATING HOURS	

SLEEP			
TO BED		HOURS	
WOKE UP		SLEPT	

EXERCISE		QUALITY			
TIME		TYPE		DURATION	

MEAL / SNACK	TIME	CALORIES
	TOTAL	

ENERGY LEVEL	NOTES
☆☆☆☆☆ ☆☆☆☆☆	

WATER INTAKE (GLASSES)

⬦ ⬦ ⬦ ⬦
⬦ ⬦ ⬦ ⬦

"It does not matter how slowly you go as long as you do not stop."
-Confucious

Intermittent Fasting Tracker

DAY		DATE		FASTING DAY	Y N	WEIGHT	

FIRST BITE		FASTING HOURS	
LAST BITE		EATING HOURS	

SLEEP

TO BED		HOURS	
WOKE UP		SLEPT	

EXERCISE   QUALITY

TIME		TYPE		DURATION	

MEAL / SNACK	TIME	CALORIES
		TOTAL

ENERGY LEVEL	NOTES
☆☆☆☆☆ ☆☆☆☆☆	

WATER INTAKE (GLASSES)

◊ ◊ ◊ ◊
◊ ◊ ◊ ◊

*"If it is important to you,
you will find a way. If
not, you'll find an excuse."
-Unknown*

Intermittent Fasting Tracker

DAY		DATE		FASTING DAY	Y N	WEIGHT	

FIRST BITE			FASTING HOURS	
LAST BITE			EATING HOURS	

SLEEP				
TO BED			HOURS	
WOKE UP			SLEPT	

EXERCISE			QUALITY	
TIME		TYPE		DURATION

MEAL / SNACK	TIME	CALORIES
	TOTAL	

ENERGY LEVEL	NOTES
☆☆☆☆☆ ☆☆☆☆☆	

WATER INTAKE (GLASSES)

◊ ◊ ◊ ◊
◊ ◊ ◊ ◊

"It does not matter how slowly you go as long as you do not stop."
-Confucious

Intermittent Fasting Tracker

DAY		DATE		FASTING DAY	Y N	WEIGHT

FIRST BITE		FASTING HOURS	
LAST BITE		EATING HOURS	

SLEEP

TO BED		HOURS	
WOKE UP		SLEPT	

EXERCISE | **QUALITY**

TIME		TYPE		DURATION	

MEAL / SNACK	TIME	CALORIES
	TOTAL	

ENERGY LEVEL	NOTES
☆☆☆☆☆	
☆☆☆☆☆	

WATER INTAKE (GLASSES)

◇◇◇◇
◇◇◇◇

"If it is important to you, you will find a way. If not, you'll find an excuse."
-Unknown

Intermittent Fasting Tracker

DAY		DATE		FASTING DAY	Y N	WEIGHT	
FIRST BITE			FASTING HOURS				
LAST BITE			EATING HOURS				

SLEEP				
TO BED		HOURS		
WOKE UP		SLEPT		

EXERCISE			QUALITY	
TIME		TYPE		DURATION

MEAL / SNACK	TIME	CALORIES
	TOTAL	

ENERGY LEVEL	NOTES
☆☆☆☆☆ ☆☆☆☆☆	

WATER INTAKE (GLASSES)

◯ ◯ ◯ ◯
◯ ◯ ◯ ◯

"It does not matter how slowly you go as long as you do not stop."
-Confucious

Intermittent Fasting Tracker

DAY		DATE		FASTING DAY	Y N	WEIGHT

FIRST BITE		FASTING HOURS	
LAST BITE		EATING HOURS	

SLEEP

TO BED		HOURS	
WOKE UP		SLEPT	

EXERCISE   QUALITY

TIME		TYPE		DURATION	

MEAL / SNACK	TIME	CALORIES
	TOTAL	

ENERGY LEVEL	NOTES
☆ ☆ ☆ ☆ ☆ ☆ ☆ ☆ ☆ ☆	
WATER INTAKE (GLASSES) ⬡ ⬡ ⬡ ⬡ ⬡ ⬡ ⬡ ⬡	

"If it is important to you, you will find a way. If not, you'll find an excuse."
-Unknown

Intermittent Fasting Tracker

DAY		DATE		FASTING DAY	Y N	WEIGHT	

FIRST BITE		FASTING HOURS	
LAST BITE		EATING HOURS	

SLEEP			
TO BED		HOURS	
WOKE UP		SLEPT	

EXERCISE		QUALITY	
TIME		TYPE		DURATION	

MEAL / SNACK	TIME	CALORIES
	TOTAL	

ENERGY LEVEL

☆☆☆☆☆

☆☆☆☆☆

WATER INTAKE (GLASSES)

◊ ◊ ◊ ◊

◊ ◊ ◊ ◊

NOTES

"It does not matter how slowly you go as long as you do not stop."
-Confucious

Intermittent Fasting Tracker

DAY		DATE		FASTING DAY	Y N	WEIGHT

FIRST BITE		FASTING HOURS	
LAST BITE		EATING HOURS	

SLEEP

TO BED		HOURS	
WOKE UP		SLEPT	

EXERCISE QUALITY

TIME		TYPE		DURATION	

MEAL / SNACK	TIME	CALORIES
	TOTAL	

ENERGY LEVEL

☆☆☆☆☆
☆☆☆☆☆

WATER INTAKE (GLASSES)

⬭⬭⬭⬭
⬭⬭⬭⬭

NOTES

"If it is important to you, you will find a way. If not, you'll find an excuse."
-Unknown

Intermittent Fasting Tracker

DAY		DATE		FASTING DAY	Y N	WEIGHT	
FIRST BITE			FASTING HOURS				
LAST BITE			EATING HOURS				

SLEEP				
TO BED		HOURS		
WOKE UP		SLEPT		

EXERCISE		QUALITY		
TIME		TYPE	DURATION	

MEAL / SNACK	TIME	CALORIES
	TOTAL	

ENERGY LEVEL	NOTES
☆☆☆☆☆	
☆☆☆☆☆	

WATER INTAKE (GLASSES)

◇◇◇◇
◇◇◇◇

"It does not matter how slowly you go as long as you do not stop."
-Confucious

Intermittent Fasting Tracker

DAY		DATE		FASTING DAY	Y N	WEIGHT

FIRST BITE		FASTING HOURS	
LAST BITE		EATING HOURS	

SLEEP

TO BED		HOURS	
WOKE UP		SLEPT	

EXERCISE QUALITY

TIME		TYPE		DURATION	

MEAL / SNACK	TIME	CALORIES
	TOTAL	

ENERGY LEVEL

☆☆☆☆☆
☆☆☆☆☆

WATER INTAKE (GLASSES)

◊◊◊◊
◊◊◊◊

NOTES

"If it is important to you,
you will find a way. If
not, you'll find an excuse."
-Unknown

Intermittent Fasting Tracker

DAY		DATE		FASTING DAY	Y N	WEIGHT	
FIRST BITE				FASTING HOURS			
LAST BITE				EATING HOURS			

SLEEP					
TO BED			HOURS		
WOKE UP			SLEPT		

EXERCISE			QUALITY		
TIME		TYPE		DURATION	

MEAL / SNACK	TIME	CALORIES
	TOTAL	

ENERGY LEVEL	NOTES
☆☆☆☆☆	
☆☆☆☆☆	

WATER INTAKE (GLASSES)

⬤ ⬤ ⬤ ⬤
⬤ ⬤ ⬤ ⬤

"It does not matter how slowly you go as long as you do not stop."
-Confucious

Intermittent Fasting Tracker

DAY		DATE		FASTING DAY	Y N	WEIGHT	

FIRST BITE		FASTING HOURS	
LAST BITE		EATING HOURS	

SLEEP			
TO BED		HOURS	
WOKE UP		SLEPT	

EXERCISE		QUALITY			
TIME		TYPE		DURATION	

MEAL / SNACK	TIME	CALORIES
		TOTAL

ENERGY LEVEL	NOTES
☆☆☆☆☆ ☆☆☆☆☆	

WATER INTAKE (GLASSES)

○○○○
○○○○

"If it is important to you, you will find a way. If not, you'll find an excuse."
-Unknown

Intermittent Fasting Tracker

DAY		DATE		FASTING DAY	Y N	WEIGHT	

FIRST BITE		FASTING HOURS	
LAST BITE		EATING HOURS	

SLEEP

TO BED		HOURS	
WOKE UP		SLEPT	

EXERCISE | | | | QUALITY

TIME		TYPE		DURATION	

MEAL / SNACK	TIME	CALORIES
	TOTAL	

ENERGY LEVEL

☆☆☆☆☆
☆☆☆☆☆

NOTES

WATER INTAKE (GLASSES)

◊ ◊ ◊ ◊
◊ ◊ ◊ ◊

"It does not matter how slowly you go as long as you do not stop."
-Confucious

Intermittent Fasting Tracker

DAY		DATE		FASTING DAY	Y N	WEIGHT	

FIRST BITE		FASTING HOURS	
LAST BITE		EATING HOURS	

SLEEP			
TO BED		HOURS	
WOKE UP		SLEPT	

EXERCISE		QUALITY		
TIME		TYPE		DURATION

MEAL / SNACK	TIME	CALORIES
	TOTAL	

ENERGY LEVEL

☆☆☆☆☆
☆☆☆☆☆

WATER INTAKE (GLASSES)

⬤⬤⬤⬤
⬤⬤⬤⬤

NOTES

"If it is important to you, you will find a way. If not, you'll find an excuse."
-Unknown

Intermittent Fasting Tracker

DAY		DATE		FASTING DAY	Y N	WEIGHT	

FIRST BITE		FASTING HOURS	
LAST BITE		EATING HOURS	

SLEEP

TO BED		HOURS	
WOKE UP		SLEPT	

EXERCISE QUALITY

TIME		TYPE		DURATION	

MEAL / SNACK	TIME	CALORIES
	TOTAL	

ENERGY LEVEL	NOTES
☆☆☆☆☆ ☆☆☆☆☆	

WATER INTAKE (GLASSES)

◊ ◊ ◊ ◊
◊ ◊ ◊ ◊

"It does not matter how slowly you go as long as you do not stop."
-Confucious

Intermittent Fasting Tracker

DAY		DATE		FASTING DAY	Y N	WEIGHT

FIRST BITE		FASTING HOURS	
LAST BITE		EATING HOURS	

SLEEP

TO BED		HOURS	
WOKE UP		SLEPT	

EXERCISE | QUALITY

TIME		TYPE		DURATION	

MEAL / SNACK	TIME	CALORIES
	TOTAL	

ENERGY LEVEL

☆☆☆☆☆
☆☆☆☆☆

WATER INTAKE (GLASSES)

🌢🌢🌢🌢
🌢🌢🌢🌢

NOTES

"If it is important to you,
you will find a way. If
not, you'll find an excuse."
-Unknown

Intermittent Fasting Tracker

DAY		DATE		FASTING DAY	Y N	WEIGHT	

FIRST BITE		FASTING HOURS	
LAST BITE		EATING HOURS	

SLEEP

TO BED		HOURS	
WOKE UP		SLEPT	

EXERCISE **QUALITY**

TIME		TYPE		DURATION	

MEAL / SNACK	TIME	CALORIES
	TOTAL	

ENERGY LEVEL	NOTES
☆☆☆☆☆ ☆☆☆☆☆	

WATER INTAKE (GLASSES)

◊ ◊ ◊ ◊
◊ ◊ ◊ ◊

"It does not matter how slowly you go as long as you do not stop."
-Confucious

Intermittent Fasting Tracker

DAY		DATE		FASTING DAY	Y N	WEIGHT	

FIRST BITE		FASTING HOURS	
LAST BITE		EATING HOURS	

SLEEP			
TO BED		HOURS	
WOKE UP		SLEPT	

EXERCISE		QUALITY	
TIME		TYPE		DURATION	

MEAL / SNACK	TIME	CALORIES
	TOTAL	

ENERGY LEVEL	NOTES
☆☆☆☆☆ ☆☆☆☆☆	

WATER INTAKE (GLASSES)

⬡ ⬡ ⬡ ⬡
⬡ ⬡ ⬡ ⬡

"If it is important to you, you will find a way. If not, you'll find an excuse."
-Unknown

Intermittent Fasting Tracker

DAY		DATE		FASTING DAY	Y N	WEIGHT	

FIRST BITE		FASTING HOURS	
LAST BITE		EATING HOURS	

SLEEP

TO BED		HOURS	
WOKE UP		SLEPT	

EXERCISE — QUALITY

TIME		TYPE		DURATION	

MEAL / SNACK	TIME	CALORIES
	TOTAL	

ENERGY LEVEL

☆☆☆☆☆
☆☆☆☆☆

WATER INTAKE (GLASSES)

◊ ◊ ◊ ◊
◊ ◊ ◊ ◊

NOTES

"It does not matter how slowly you go as long as you do not stop."
-Confucious

Intermittent Fasting Tracker

DAY		DATE		FASTING DAY	Y N	WEIGHT

FIRST BITE		FASTING HOURS	
LAST BITE		EATING HOURS	

SLEEP

TO BED		HOURS	
WOKE UP		SLEPT	

EXERCISE QUALITY

TIME		TYPE		DURATION	

MEAL / SNACK	TIME	CALORIES
	TOTAL	

ENERGY LEVEL

☆☆☆☆☆
☆☆☆☆☆

WATER INTAKE (GLASSES)

◊ ◊ ◊ ◊
◊ ◊ ◊ ◊

NOTES

"If it is important to you, you will find a way. If not, you'll find an excuse."
-Unknown

Intermittent Fasting Tracker

DAY		DATE		FASTING DAY	Y N	WEIGHT	

FIRST BITE			FASTING HOURS	
LAST BITE			EATING HOURS	

SLEEP

TO BED			HOURS	
WOKE UP			SLEPT	

EXERCISE QUALITY

TIME		TYPE		DURATION	

MEAL / SNACK	TIME	CALORIES
		TOTAL

ENERGY LEVEL	NOTES
☆☆☆☆☆	
☆☆☆☆☆	

WATER INTAKE (GLASSES)

◯ ◯ ◯ ◯
◯ ◯ ◯ ◯

"It does not matter how slowly you go as long as you do not stop."
-Confucious

Intermittent Fasting Tracker

DAY		DATE		FASTING DAY	Y N	WEIGHT	

FIRST BITE		FASTING HOURS	
LAST BITE		EATING HOURS	

SLEEP

TO BED		HOURS	
WOKE UP		SLEPT	

EXERCISE   QUALITY

TIME		TYPE		DURATION	

MEAL / SNACK	TIME	CALORIES
	TOTAL	

ENERGY LEVEL	NOTES
☆☆☆☆☆ ☆☆☆☆☆	

WATER INTAKE (GLASSES)

⬯ ⬯ ⬯ ⬯
⬯ ⬯ ⬯ ⬯

"If it is important to you, you will find a way. If not, you'll find an excuse."
-Unknown

Intermittent Fasting Tracker

DAY		DATE		FASTING DAY	Y N	WEIGHT	

FIRST BITE		FASTING HOURS	
LAST BITE		EATING HOURS	

SLEEP

TO BED		HOURS	
WOKE UP		SLEPT	

EXERCISE   QUALITY

TIME		TYPE		DURATION	

MEAL / SNACK	TIME	CALORIES
	TOTAL	

ENERGY LEVEL

☆☆☆☆☆
☆☆☆☆☆

WATER INTAKE (GLASSES)

○○○○
○○○○

NOTES

"It does not matter how slowly you go as long as you do not stop."
-Confucious

Intermittent Fasting Tracker

DAY		DATE		FASTING DAY	Y N	WEIGHT	

FIRST BITE		FASTING HOURS	
LAST BITE		EATING HOURS	

SLEEP

TO BED		HOURS	
WOKE UP		SLEPT	

EXERCISE   **QUALITY**

TIME		TYPE		DURATION	

MEAL / SNACK	TIME	CALORIES
	TOTAL	

ENERGY LEVEL	NOTES
☆☆☆☆☆	
☆☆☆☆☆	

WATER INTAKE (GLASSES)

◇ ◇ ◇ ◇
◇ ◇ ◇ ◇

"If it is important to you,
you will find a way. If
not, you'll find an excuse."
-Unknown

Intermittent Fasting Tracker

DAY		DATE		FASTING DAY	Y N	WEIGHT	

FIRST BITE		FASTING HOURS	
LAST BITE		EATING HOURS	

SLEEP

TO BED		HOURS	
WOKE UP		SLEPT	

EXERCISE — QUALITY

TIME		TYPE		DURATION	

MEAL / SNACK	TIME	CALORIES
	TOTAL	

ENERGY LEVEL

☆☆☆☆☆
☆☆☆☆☆

WATER INTAKE (GLASSES)

◊ ◊ ◊ ◊
◊ ◊ ◊ ◊

NOTES

"It does not matter how slowly you go as long as you do not stop."
-Confucious

Intermittent Fasting Tracker

DAY		DATE		FASTING DAY	Y N	WEIGHT	

FIRST BITE		FASTING HOURS	
LAST BITE		EATING HOURS	

SLEEP

TO BED		HOURS	
WOKE UP		SLEPT	

EXERCISE QUALITY

TIME		TYPE		DURATION	

MEAL / SNACK	TIME	CALORIES
		TOTAL

ENERGY LEVEL	NOTES
☆☆☆☆☆	
☆☆☆☆☆	

WATER INTAKE (GLASSES)

◊◊◊◊
◊◊◊◊

"If it is important to you, you will find a way. If not, you'll find an excuse."
-Unknown

Intermittent Fasting Tracker

DAY		DATE		FASTING DAY	Y N	WEIGHT	

FIRST BITE			FASTING HOURS	
LAST BITE			EATING HOURS	

SLEEP

TO BED		HOURS	
WOKE UP		SLEPT	

EXERCISE		QUALITY	
TIME		TYPE		DURATION	

MEAL / SNACK	TIME	CALORIES
	TOTAL	

ENERGY LEVEL	NOTES

☆☆☆☆☆
☆☆☆☆☆

WATER INTAKE (GLASSES)

⬯⬯⬯⬯
⬯⬯⬯⬯

"It does not matter how slowly you go as long as you do not stop."
-Confucious

Intermittent Fasting Tracker

DAY		DATE		FASTING DAY	Y N	WEIGHT	

FIRST BITE		FASTING HOURS	
LAST BITE		EATING HOURS	

SLEEP

TO BED		HOURS	
WOKE UP		SLEPT	

EXERCISE QUALITY

TIME		TYPE		DURATION	

MEAL / SNACK	TIME	CALORIES
		TOTAL

ENERGY LEVEL

☆☆☆☆☆
☆☆☆☆☆

NOTES

WATER INTAKE (GLASSES)

○○○○
○○○○

*"If it is important to you,
you will find a way. If
not, you'll find an excuse."
-Unknown*

Intermittent Fasting Tracker

DAY		DATE		FASTING DAY	Y N	WEIGHT	
FIRST BITE			FASTING HOURS				
LAST BITE			EATING HOURS				

SLEEP					
TO BED			HOURS		
WOKE UP			SLEPT		

EXERCISE			QUALITY		
TIME		TYPE		DURATION	

MEAL / SNACK	TIME	CALORIES
	TOTAL	

ENERGY LEVEL	NOTES
☆☆☆☆☆	
☆☆☆☆☆	

WATER INTAKE (GLASSES)

◇◇◇◇
◇◇◇◇

"It does not matter how slowly you go as long as you do not stop."
-Confucious

Intermittent Fasting Tracker

DAY		DATE		FASTING DAY	Y N	WEIGHT

FIRST BITE		FASTING HOURS	
LAST BITE		EATING HOURS	

SLEEP

TO BED		HOURS	
WOKE UP		SLEPT	

EXERCISE   QUALITY

TIME		TYPE		DURATION	

MEAL / SNACK	TIME	CALORIES
	TOTAL	

ENERGY LEVEL	NOTES
☆☆☆☆☆ ☆☆☆☆☆	

WATER INTAKE (GLASSES)

◯ ◯ ◯ ◯
◯ ◯ ◯ ◯

"If it is important to you,
you will find a way. If
not, you'll find an excuse."
-Unknown

Intermittent Fasting Tracker

DAY		DATE		FASTING DAY	Y N	WEIGHT	

FIRST BITE		FASTING HOURS	
LAST BITE		EATING HOURS	

SLEEP			
TO BED		HOURS	
WOKE UP		SLEPT	

EXERCISE		QUALITY	
TIME		TYPE	DURATION

MEAL / SNACK	TIME	CALORIES
	TOTAL	

ENERGY LEVEL

☆☆☆☆☆
☆☆☆☆☆

WATER INTAKE (GLASSES)

◇ ◇ ◇ ◇
◇ ◇ ◇ ◇

NOTES

"It does not matter how slowly you go as long as you do not stop."
-Confucious

Intermittent Fasting Tracker

DAY		DATE		FASTING DAY	Y N	WEIGHT

FIRST BITE		FASTING HOURS	
LAST BITE		EATING HOURS	

SLEEP			
TO BED		HOURS	
WOKE UP		SLEPT	

EXERCISE		QUALITY	
TIME		TYPE		DURATION	

MEAL / SNACK	TIME	CALORIES
		TOTAL

ENERGY LEVEL	NOTES
☆☆☆☆☆	
☆☆☆☆☆	

WATER INTAKE (GLASSES)

⬦⬦⬦⬦
⬦⬦⬦⬦

"If it is important to you, you will find a way. If not, you'll find an excuse."
-Unknown

Intermittent Fasting Tracker

DAY		DATE		FASTING DAY	Y N	WEIGHT	

FIRST BITE		FASTING HOURS	
LAST BITE		EATING HOURS	

SLEEP

TO BED		HOURS	
WOKE UP		SLEPT	

EXERCISE			QUALITY	
TIME		TYPE		DURATION

MEAL / SNACK	TIME	CALORIES
	TOTAL	

ENERGY LEVEL	NOTES
☆☆☆☆☆	
☆☆☆☆☆	

WATER INTAKE (GLASSES)

○○○○
○○○○

"It does not matter how slowly you go as long as you do not stop."
-Confucious

Intermittent Fasting Tracker

DAY		DATE		FASTING DAY	Y N	WEIGHT	

FIRST BITE		FASTING HOURS	
LAST BITE		EATING HOURS	

SLEEP

TO BED		HOURS	
WOKE UP		SLEPT	

EXERCISE   QUALITY

TIME		TYPE		DURATION	

MEAL / SNACK	TIME	CALORIES
		TOTAL

ENERGY LEVEL	NOTES
☆ ☆ ☆ ☆ ☆	
☆ ☆ ☆ ☆ ☆	
WATER INTAKE (GLASSES)	
⬦ ⬦ ⬦ ⬦ ⬦ ⬦ ⬦ ⬦	

"If it is important to you,
you will find a way. If
not, you'll find an excuse."
-Unknown

Intermittent Fasting Tracker

DAY		DATE		FASTING DAY	Y N	WEIGHT	

FIRST BITE			FASTING HOURS	
LAST BITE			EATING HOURS	

SLEEP				
TO BED			HOURS	
WOKE UP			SLEPT	

EXERCISE		QUALITY		
TIME		TYPE	DURATION	

MEAL / SNACK	TIME	CALORIES
	TOTAL	

ENERGY LEVEL	NOTES
☆☆☆☆☆	
☆☆☆☆☆	

WATER INTAKE (GLASSES)

◊ ◊ ◊ ◊
◊ ◊ ◊ ◊

"It does not matter how slowly you go as long as you do not stop."
-Confucious

Intermittent Fasting Tracker

DAY		DATE		FASTING DAY	Y N	WEIGHT

FIRST BITE		FASTING HOURS	
LAST BITE		EATING HOURS	

SLEEP

TO BED		HOURS	
WOKE UP		SLEPT	

EXERCISE   **QUALITY**

TIME		TYPE		DURATION	

MEAL / SNACK	TIME	CALORIES
	TOTAL	

ENERGY LEVEL   **NOTES**

☆☆☆☆☆

☆☆☆☆☆

WATER INTAKE (GLASSES)

⬡⬡⬡⬡

⬡⬡⬡⬡

*"If it is important to you,
you will find a way. If
not, you'll find an excuse."*
-Unknown

Intermittent Fasting Tracker

DAY		DATE		FASTING DAY	Y N	WEIGHT	

FIRST BITE		FASTING HOURS	
LAST BITE		EATING HOURS	

SLEEP

TO BED		HOURS	
WOKE UP		SLEPT	

EXERCISE — **QUALITY**

TIME		TYPE		DURATION	

MEAL / SNACK	TIME	CALORIES
		TOTAL

ENERGY LEVEL

☆☆☆☆☆
☆☆☆☆☆

WATER INTAKE (GLASSES)

◇◇◇◇
◇◇◇◇

NOTES

"It does not matter how slowly you go as long as you do not stop."
-Confucious

Intermittent Fasting Tracker

DAY		DATE		FASTING DAY	Y N	WEIGHT	
FIRST BITE			FASTING HOURS				
LAST BITE			EATING HOURS				

SLEEP				
TO BED		HOURS		
WOKE UP		SLEPT		

EXERCISE		QUALITY		
TIME		TYPE		DURATION

MEAL / SNACK	TIME	CALORIES
		TOTAL

ENERGY LEVEL

☆☆☆☆☆
☆☆☆☆☆

WATER INTAKE (GLASSES)

◊ ◊ ◊ ◊
◊ ◊ ◊ ◊

NOTES

"If it is important to you, you will find a way. If not, you'll find an excuse."
-Unknown

Intermittent Fasting Tracker

DAY		DATE		FASTING DAY	Y N	WEIGHT	

FIRST BITE		FASTING HOURS	
LAST BITE		EATING HOURS	

SLEEP			
TO BED		HOURS	
WOKE UP		SLEPT	

EXERCISE		QUALITY			
TIME		TYPE		DURATION	

MEAL / SNACK	TIME	CALORIES
	TOTAL	

ENERGY LEVEL

☆☆☆☆☆
☆☆☆☆☆

NOTES

WATER INTAKE (GLASSES)

⬤⬤⬤⬤
⬤⬤⬤⬤

"It does not matter how slowly you go as long as you do not stop."
-Confucious

Intermittent Fasting Tracker

DAY		DATE		FASTING DAY	Y N	WEIGHT

FIRST BITE		FASTING HOURS	
LAST BITE		EATING HOURS	

SLEEP

TO BED		HOURS	
WOKE UP		SLEPT	

EXERCISE   QUALITY

TIME		TYPE		DURATION	

MEAL / SNACK	TIME	CALORIES
	TOTAL	

ENERGY LEVEL

☆☆☆☆☆
☆☆☆☆☆

WATER INTAKE (GLASSES)

◊ ◊ ◊ ◊
◊ ◊ ◊ ◊

NOTES

"If it is important to you,
you will find a way. If
not, you'll find an excuse."
-Unknown

Intermittent Fasting Tracker

DAY		DATE		FASTING DAY	Y N	WEIGHT	
FIRST BITE			FASTING HOURS				
LAST BITE			EATING HOURS				

SLEEP				
TO BED		HOURS		
WOKE UP		SLEPT		

EXERCISE		QUALITY		
TIME		TYPE		DURATION

MEAL / SNACK	TIME	CALORIES
	TOTAL	

ENERGY LEVEL	NOTES
☆☆☆☆☆ ☆☆☆☆☆	

WATER INTAKE (GLASSES)

◇◇◇◇
◇◇◇◇

"It does not matter how slowly you go as long as you do not stop."
-Confucious

Intermittent Fasting Tracker

DAY		DATE		FASTING DAY	Y N	WEIGHT
FIRST BITE			FASTING HOURS			
LAST BITE			EATING HOURS			

SLEEP			
TO BED		HOURS	
WOKE UP		SLEPT	

EXERCISE		QUALITY	
TIME		TYPE		DURATION	

MEAL / SNACK	TIME	CALORIES
		TOTAL

ENERGY LEVEL	NOTES
☆☆☆☆☆	
☆☆☆☆☆	
WATER INTAKE (GLASSES)	
⬤⬤⬤⬤ ⬤⬤⬤⬤	

"If it is important to you, you will find a way. If not, you'll find an excuse."
-Unknown

Intermittent Fasting Tracker

DAY		DATE		FASTING DAY	Y N	WEIGHT	

FIRST BITE		FASTING HOURS	
LAST BITE		EATING HOURS	

SLEEP

TO BED		HOURS	
WOKE UP		SLEPT	

EXERCISE | | | **QUALITY**

TIME		TYPE		DURATION	

MEAL / SNACK	TIME	CALORIES
		TOTAL

ENERGY LEVEL

☆☆☆☆☆
☆☆☆☆☆

WATER INTAKE (GLASSES)

◊ ◊ ◊ ◊
◊ ◊ ◊ ◊

NOTES

"It does not matter how slowly you go as long as you do not stop."
-Confucious

Intermittent Fasting Tracker

DAY		DATE		FASTING DAY	Y N	WEIGHT	
FIRST BITE				FASTING HOURS			
LAST BITE				EATING HOURS			

SLEEP			
TO BED		HOURS	
WOKE UP		SLEPT	

EXERCISE			QUALITY	
TIME		TYPE		DURATION

MEAL / SNACK	TIME	CALORIES
		TOTAL

ENERGY LEVEL	NOTES
☆☆☆☆☆	
☆☆☆☆☆	
WATER INTAKE (GLASSES)	
⬥⬥⬥⬥ ⬥⬥⬥⬥	

"If it is important to you, you will find a way. If not, you'll find an excuse."
-Unknown

Intermittent Fasting Tracker

DAY		DATE		FASTING DAY	Y N	WEIGHT	

FIRST BITE			FASTING HOURS	
LAST BITE			EATING HOURS	

SLEEP

TO BED		HOURS	
WOKE UP		SLEPT	

EXERCISE QUALITY

TIME		TYPE		DURATION	

MEAL / SNACK	TIME	CALORIES
	TOTAL	

ENERGY LEVEL	NOTES
☆☆☆☆☆ ☆☆☆☆☆	

WATER INTAKE (GLASSES)

◇ ◇ ◇ ◇
◇ ◇ ◇ ◇

"It does not matter how slowly you go as long as you do not stop."
-Confucious

Intermittent Fasting Tracker

DAY		DATE		FASTING DAY	Y N	WEIGHT

FIRST BITE		FASTING HOURS	
LAST BITE		EATING HOURS	

SLEEP

TO BED		HOURS	
WOKE UP		SLEPT	

EXERCISE   QUALITY

TIME		TYPE		DURATION	

MEAL / SNACK	TIME	CALORIES
	TOTAL	

ENERGY LEVEL

☆☆☆☆☆
☆☆☆☆☆

WATER INTAKE (GLASSES)

◌◌◌◌
◌◌◌◌

NOTES

"If it is important to you, you will find a way. If not, you'll find an excuse."
-Unknown

Intermittent Fasting Tracker

DAY		DATE		FASTING DAY	Y N	WEIGHT	

FIRST BITE		FASTING HOURS	
LAST BITE		EATING HOURS	

SLEEP

TO BED		HOURS	
WOKE UP		SLEPT	

EXERCISE		QUALITY	
TIME		TYPE		DURATION	

MEAL / SNACK	TIME	CALORIES
	TOTAL	

ENERGY LEVEL

☆☆☆☆☆
☆☆☆☆☆

WATER INTAKE (GLASSES)

⬦ ⬦ ⬦ ⬦
⬦ ⬦ ⬦ ⬦

NOTES

"It does not matter how slowly you go as long as you do not stop."
-Confucious

Intermittent Fasting Tracker

DAY		DATE		FASTING DAY	Y N	WEIGHT	

FIRST BITE		FASTING HOURS	
LAST BITE		EATING HOURS	

SLEEP			
TO BED		HOURS	
WOKE UP		SLEPT	

EXERCISE		QUALITY	
TIME		TYPE	DURATION

MEAL / SNACK	TIME	CALORIES
		TOTAL

ENERGY LEVEL	NOTES
☆☆☆☆☆ ☆☆☆☆☆	

WATER INTAKE (GLASSES)

◇ ◇ ◇ ◇
◇ ◇ ◇ ◇

"If it is important to you, you will find a way. If not, you'll find an excuse."
-Unknown

Intermittent Fasting Tracker

DAY		DATE		FASTING DAY	Y N	WEIGHT	

FIRST BITE			FASTING HOURS	
LAST BITE			EATING HOURS	

SLEEP

TO BED		HOURS	
WOKE UP		SLEPT	

EXERCISE   QUALITY

TIME		TYPE		DURATION	

MEAL / SNACK	TIME	CALORIES
	TOTAL	

ENERGY LEVEL	NOTES
☆☆☆☆☆ ☆☆☆☆☆	

WATER INTAKE (GLASSES)

⬭⬭⬭⬭
⬭⬭⬭⬭

"It does not matter how slowly you go as long as you do not stop."
-Confucious

Intermittent Fasting Tracker

DAY		DATE		FASTING DAY	Y N	WEIGHT	
FIRST BITE				FASTING HOURS			
LAST BITE				EATING HOURS			

SLEEP				
TO BED			HOURS	
WOKE UP			SLEPT	

EXERCISE			QUALITY	
TIME		TYPE		DURATION

MEAL / SNACK	TIME	CALORIES
	TOTAL	

ENERGY LEVEL

☆☆☆☆☆

☆☆☆☆☆

WATER INTAKE (GLASSES)

◯◯◯◯
◯◯◯◯

NOTES

"If it is important to you, you will find a way. If not, you'll find an excuse."
-Unknown

Intermittent Fasting Tracker

DAY		DATE		FASTING DAY	Y N	WEIGHT

FIRST BITE		FASTING HOURS	
LAST BITE		EATING HOURS	

SLEEP

TO BED		HOURS	
WOKE UP		SLEPT	

EXERCISE   QUALITY

TIME		TYPE		DURATION	

MEAL / SNACK	TIME	CALORIES
		TOTAL

ENERGY LEVEL

☆☆☆☆☆
☆☆☆☆☆

WATER INTAKE (GLASSES)

◯◯◯◯
◯◯◯◯

NOTES

"It does not matter how slowly you go as long as you do not stop."
-Confucious

Intermittent Fasting Tracker

DAY		DATE		FASTING DAY	Y N	WEIGHT	

FIRST BITE		FASTING HOURS	
LAST BITE		EATING HOURS	

SLEEP			
TO BED		HOURS	
WOKE UP		SLEPT	

EXERCISE		QUALITY	
TIME		TYPE		DURATION	

MEAL / SNACK	TIME	CALORIES
	TOTAL	

ENERGY LEVEL

☆☆☆☆☆
☆☆☆☆☆

WATER INTAKE (GLASSES)

◇◇◇◇
◇◇◇◇

NOTES

"If it is important to you, you will find a way. If not, you'll find an excuse."
-Unknown

Intermittent Fasting Tracker

| DAY | | DATE | | FASTING DAY | Y N | WEIGHT | |

| FIRST BITE | | FASTING HOURS | |
| LAST BITE | | EATING HOURS | |

SLEEP

| TO BED | | HOURS | |
| WOKE UP | | SLEPT | |

EXERCISE   QUALITY

| TIME | | TYPE | | DURATION | |

MEAL / SNACK	TIME	CALORIES
	TOTAL	

ENERGY LEVEL	NOTES

☆☆☆☆☆
☆☆☆☆☆

WATER INTAKE (GLASSES)

⬯ ⬯ ⬯ ⬯
⬯ ⬯ ⬯ ⬯

"It does not matter how slowly you go as long as you do not stop."
-Confucious

Intermittent Fasting Tracker

DAY		DATE		FASTING DAY	Y N	WEIGHT	

FIRST BITE			FASTING HOURS	
LAST BITE			EATING HOURS	

SLEEP				
TO BED			HOURS	
WOKE UP			SLEPT	

EXERCISE			QUALITY	
TIME		TYPE		DURATION

MEAL / SNACK	TIME	CALORIES
		TOTAL

ENERGY LEVEL	NOTES
☆☆☆☆☆	
☆☆☆☆☆	

WATER INTAKE (GLASSES)

◌ ◌ ◌ ◌
◌ ◌ ◌ ◌

"If it is important to you,
you will find a way. If
not, you'll find an excuse."
-Unknown

Intermittent Fasting Tracker

DAY		DATE		FASTING DAY	Y N	WEIGHT	

FIRST BITE		FASTING HOURS	
LAST BITE		EATING HOURS	

SLEEP

TO BED		HOURS	
WOKE UP		SLEPT	

EXERCISE QUALITY

TIME		TYPE		DURATION	

MEAL / SNACK	TIME	CALORIES
	TOTAL	

ENERGY LEVEL

☆☆☆☆☆
☆☆☆☆☆

WATER INTAKE (GLASSES)

◯◯◯◯
◯◯◯◯

NOTES

"It does not matter how slowly you go as long as you do not stop."
-Confucious

Intermittent Fasting Tracker

DAY		DATE		FASTING DAY	Y N	WEIGHT

FIRST BITE		FASTING HOURS	
LAST BITE		EATING HOURS	

SLEEP

TO BED		HOURS	
WOKE UP		SLEPT	

EXERCISE   **QUALITY**

TIME		TYPE		DURATION	

MEAL / SNACK	TIME	CALORIES
	TOTAL	

ENERGY LEVEL

☆ ☆ ☆ ☆ ☆
☆ ☆ ☆ ☆ ☆

WATER INTAKE (GLASSES)

◯ ◯ ◯ ◯
◯ ◯ ◯ ◯

NOTES

*"If it is important to you,
you will find a way. If
not, you'll find an excuse."
-Unknown*

Intermittent Fasting Tracker

DAY		DATE		FASTING DAY	Y N	WEIGHT	
FIRST BITE			FASTING HOURS				
LAST BITE			EATING HOURS				

SLEEP				
TO BED		HOURS		
WOKE UP		SLEPT		

EXERCISE		QUALITY			
TIME		TYPE		DURATION	

MEAL / SNACK	TIME	CALORIES
	TOTAL	

ENERGY LEVEL

☆☆☆☆☆
☆☆☆☆☆

WATER INTAKE (GLASSES)

◌ ◌ ◌ ◌
◌ ◌ ◌ ◌

NOTES

"It does not matter how slowly you go as long as you do not stop."
-Confucious

Intermittent Fasting Tracker

DAY		DATE		FASTING DAY	Y N	WEIGHT	

FIRST BITE		FASTING HOURS	
LAST BITE		EATING HOURS	

SLEEP

TO BED		HOURS	
WOKE UP		SLEPT	

EXERCISE — QUALITY

TIME		TYPE		DURATION	

MEAL / SNACK	TIME	CALORIES
		TOTAL

ENERGY LEVEL

☆☆☆☆☆
☆☆☆☆☆

WATER INTAKE (GLASSES)

◊◊◊◊
◊◊◊◊

NOTES

"If it is important to you.
you will find a way. If
not. you'll find an excuse."
-Unknown

Intermittent Fasting Tracker

DAY		DATE		FASTING DAY	Y N	WEIGHT	

FIRST BITE		FASTING HOURS	
LAST BITE		EATING HOURS	

SLEEP

TO BED		HOURS	
WOKE UP		SLEPT	

EXERCISE   QUALITY

TIME		TYPE		DURATION	

MEAL / SNACK	TIME	CALORIES
	TOTAL	

ENERGY LEVEL

☆☆☆☆☆
☆☆☆☆☆

WATER INTAKE (GLASSES)

◌ ◌ ◌ ◌
◌ ◌ ◌ ◌

NOTES

"It does not matter how slowly you go as long as you do not stop."
-Confucious

Intermittent Fasting Tracker

DAY		DATE		FASTING DAY	Y N	WEIGHT

FIRST BITE		FASTING HOURS	
LAST BITE		EATING HOURS	

SLEEP

TO BED		HOURS	
WOKE UP		SLEPT	

EXERCISE | QUALITY

TIME		TYPE		DURATION	

MEAL / SNACK	TIME	CALORIES
		TOTAL

ENERGY LEVEL

☆☆☆☆☆
☆☆☆☆☆

WATER INTAKE (GLASSES)

◯◯◯◯
◯◯◯◯

NOTES

*"If it is important to you.
you will find a way. If
not. you'll find an excuse."*
-Unknown

Intermittent Fasting Tracker

DAY		DATE		FASTING DAY	Y N	WEIGHT	
FIRST BITE			FASTING HOURS				
LAST BITE			EATING HOURS				

SLEEP				
TO BED		HOURS		
WOKE UP		SLEPT		

EXERCISE		QUALITY		
TIME		TYPE		DURATION

MEAL / SNACK	TIME	CALORIES
	TOTAL	

ENERGY LEVEL	NOTES
☆☆☆☆☆ ☆☆☆☆☆	

WATER INTAKE (GLASSES)

◯ ◯ ◯ ◯
◯ ◯ ◯ ◯

"It does not matter how slowly you go as long as you do not stop."
-Confucious

Intermittent Fasting Tracker

DAY		DATE		FASTING DAY	Y N	WEIGHT	

FIRST BITE		FASTING HOURS	
LAST BITE		EATING HOURS	

SLEEP			
TO BED		HOURS	
WOKE UP		SLEPT	

EXERCISE		QUALITY	
TIME		TYPE		DURATION	

MEAL / SNACK	TIME	CALORIES
	TOTAL	

ENERGY LEVEL	NOTES
☆☆☆☆☆	
☆☆☆☆☆	

WATER INTAKE (GLASSES)

◯ ◯ ◯ ◯
◯ ◯ ◯ ◯

*"If it is important to you,
you will find a way. If
not, you'll find an excuse."
-Unknown*

Intermittent Fasting Tracker

DAY		DATE		FASTING DAY	Y N	WEIGHT	

FIRST BITE		FASTING HOURS	
LAST BITE		EATING HOURS	

SLEEP

TO BED		HOURS	
WOKE UP		SLEPT	

EXERCISE   **QUALITY**

TIME		TYPE		DURATION	

MEAL / SNACK	TIME	CALORIES
	TOTAL	

ENERGY LEVEL

☆☆☆☆☆
☆☆☆☆☆

WATER INTAKE (GLASSES)

◊ ◊ ◊ ◊
◊ ◊ ◊ ◊

NOTES

"It does not matter how slowly you go as long as you do not stop."
-Confucious

Intermittent Fasting Tracker

DAY		DATE		FASTING DAY	Y N	WEIGHT	

FIRST BITE		FASTING HOURS	
LAST BITE		EATING HOURS	

SLEEP

TO BED		HOURS	
WOKE UP		SLEPT	

EXERCISE · **QUALITY**

TIME		TYPE		DURATION	

MEAL / SNACK	TIME	CALORIES
		TOTAL

ENERGY LEVEL

☆☆☆☆☆
☆☆☆☆☆

WATER INTAKE (GLASSES)

◊ ◊ ◊ ◊
◊ ◊ ◊ ◊

NOTES

"If it is important to you, you will find a way. If not, you'll find an excuse."
-Unknown

Intermittent Fasting Tracker

DAY		DATE		FASTING DAY	Y N	WEIGHT	
FIRST BITE			FASTING HOURS				
LAST BITE			EATING HOURS				

SLEEP				
TO BED		HOURS		
WOKE UP		SLEPT		

EXERCISE			QUALITY		
TIME		TYPE		DURATION	

MEAL / SNACK	TIME	CALORIES
	TOTAL	

ENERGY LEVEL	NOTES
☆☆☆☆☆ ☆☆☆☆☆	

WATER INTAKE (GLASSES)

◇ ◇ ◇ ◇
◇ ◇ ◇ ◇

"It does not matter how slowly you go as long as you do not stop."
-Confucious

Intermittent Fasting Tracker

DAY		DATE		FASTING DAY	Y N	WEIGHT	

FIRST BITE		FASTING HOURS	
LAST BITE		EATING HOURS	

SLEEP			
TO BED		HOURS	
WOKE UP		SLEPT	

EXERCISE		QUALITY	
TIME		TYPE		DURATION	

MEAL / SNACK	TIME	CALORIES
		TOTAL

ENERGY LEVEL

☆☆☆☆☆

☆☆☆☆☆

WATER INTAKE (GLASSES)

◌ ◌ ◌ ◌

◌ ◌ ◌ ◌

NOTES

"If it is important to you, you will find a way. If not, you'll find an excuse."
-Unknown

Intermittent Fasting Tracker

DAY		DATE		FASTING DAY	Y N	WEIGHT	
FIRST BITE			FASTING HOURS				
LAST BITE			EATING HOURS				

SLEEP				
TO BED		HOURS		
WOKE UP		SLEPT		

EXERCISE		QUALITY			
TIME		TYPE		DURATION	

MEAL / SNACK	TIME	CALORIES
	TOTAL	

ENERGY LEVEL	NOTES
☆☆☆☆☆	
☆☆☆☆☆	

WATER INTAKE (GLASSES)

◇ ◇ ◇ ◇
◇ ◇ ◇ ◇

"It does not matter how slowly you go as long as you do not stop."
-Confucious

Intermittent Fasting Tracker

DAY		DATE		FASTING DAY	Y N	WEIGHT	

FIRST BITE		FASTING HOURS	
LAST BITE		EATING HOURS	

SLEEP			
TO BED		HOURS	
WOKE UP		SLEPT	

EXERCISE		QUALITY		
TIME		TYPE		DURATION

MEAL / SNACK	TIME	CALORIES
		TOTAL

ENERGY LEVEL	NOTES
☆☆☆☆☆ ☆☆☆☆☆	
WATER INTAKE (GLASSES)	
⬨⬨⬨⬨ ⬨⬨⬨⬨	

"If it is important to you, you will find a way. If not, you'll find an excuse."
-Unknown

Intermittent Fasting Tracker

DAY		DATE		FASTING DAY	Y N	WEIGHT	

FIRST BITE			FASTING HOURS	
LAST BITE			EATING HOURS	

SLEEP

TO BED		HOURS	
WOKE UP		SLEPT	

EXERCISE QUALITY

TIME		TYPE		DURATION	

MEAL / SNACK	TIME	CALORIES
	TOTAL	

ENERGY LEVEL

☆☆☆☆☆
☆☆☆☆☆

WATER INTAKE (GLASSES)

◊ ◊ ◊ ◊
◊ ◊ ◊ ◊

NOTES

"It does not matter how slowly you go as long as you do not stop."
-Confucious

Intermittent Fasting Tracker

DAY		DATE		FASTING DAY	Y N	WEIGHT	

FIRST BITE		FASTING HOURS	
LAST BITE		EATING HOURS	

SLEEP			
TO BED		HOURS	
WOKE UP		SLEPT	

EXERCISE		QUALITY	
TIME		TYPE		DURATION	

MEAL / SNACK	TIME	CALORIES
		TOTAL

ENERGY LEVEL

☆☆☆☆☆
☆☆☆☆☆

WATER INTAKE (GLASSES)

◯◯◯◯
◯◯◯◯

NOTES

*"If it is important to you,
you will find a way. If
not, you'll find an excuse."
-Unknown*

Intermittent Fasting Tracker

| DAY | | DATE | | FASTING DAY | Y N | WEIGHT | |

| FIRST BITE | | | FASTING HOURS | |
| LAST BITE | | | EATING HOURS | |

SLEEP				
TO BED			HOURS	
WOKE UP			SLEPT	

| EXERCISE | | | QUALITY | | |
| TIME | | TYPE | | DURATION | |

MEAL / SNACK	TIME	CALORIES
	TOTAL	

ENERGY LEVEL	NOTES
☆☆☆☆☆ ☆☆☆☆☆	

WATER INTAKE (GLASSES)

◊ ◊ ◊ ◊
◊ ◊ ◊ ◊

"It does not matter how slowly you go as long as you do not stop."
-Confucious

Intermittent Fasting Tracker

DAY		DATE		FASTING DAY	Y N	WEIGHT	

FIRST BITE		FASTING HOURS	
LAST BITE		EATING HOURS	

SLEEP

TO BED		HOURS	
WOKE UP		SLEPT	

EXERCISE | | | | **QUALITY**

TIME		TYPE		DURATION	

MEAL / SNACK	TIME	CALORIES
	TOTAL	

ENERGY LEVEL

☆☆☆☆☆
☆☆☆☆☆

NOTES

WATER INTAKE (GLASSES)

⬡⬡⬡⬡
⬡⬡⬡⬡

"If it is important to you,
you will find a way. If
not, you'll find an excuse."
-Unknown

Intermittent Fasting Tracker

DAY		DATE		FASTING DAY	Y N	WEIGHT	

FIRST BITE		FASTING HOURS	
LAST BITE		EATING HOURS	

SLEEP

TO BED		HOURS	
WOKE UP		SLEPT	

EXERCISE QUALITY

TIME		TYPE		DURATION	

MEAL / SNACK	TIME	CALORIES
	TOTAL	

ENERGY LEVEL

☆☆☆☆☆
☆☆☆☆☆

WATER INTAKE (GLASSES)

◇◇◇◇
◇◇◇◇

NOTES

"It does not matter how slowly you go as long as you do not stop."
-Confucious

Intermittent Fasting Tracker

DAY		DATE		FASTING DAY	Y N	WEIGHT	

FIRST BITE		FASTING HOURS	
LAST BITE		EATING HOURS	

SLEEP			
TO BED		HOURS	
WOKE UP		SLEPT	

EXERCISE		QUALITY	
TIME		TYPE	DURATION

MEAL / SNACK	TIME	CALORIES
	TOTAL	

ENERGY LEVEL	NOTES
☆☆☆☆☆ ☆☆☆☆☆	

WATER INTAKE (GLASSES)

◯ ◯ ◯ ◯
◯ ◯ ◯ ◯

*"If it is important to you,
you will find a way. If
not, you'll find an excuse."
-Unknown*

Intermittent Fasting Tracker

DAY		DATE		FASTING DAY	Y N	WEIGHT	

FIRST BITE		FASTING HOURS	
LAST BITE		EATING HOURS	

SLEEP

TO BED		HOURS	
WOKE UP		SLEPT	

EXERCISE QUALITY

TIME		TYPE		DURATION	

MEAL / SNACK	TIME	CALORIES
	TOTAL	

ENERGY LEVEL

☆☆☆☆☆
☆☆☆☆☆

NOTES

WATER INTAKE (GLASSES)

◇◇◇◇
◇◇◇◇

"It does not matter how slowly you go as long as you do not stop."
-Confucious

Intermittent Fasting Tracker

DAY		DATE		FASTING DAY	Y N	WEIGHT	

FIRST BITE		FASTING HOURS	
LAST BITE		EATING HOURS	

SLEEP

TO BED		HOURS	
WOKE UP		SLEPT	

EXERCISE | **QUALITY**

TIME		TYPE		DURATION	

MEAL / SNACK	TIME	CALORIES
	TOTAL	

ENERGY LEVEL	NOTES

☆ ☆ ☆ ☆ ☆
☆ ☆ ☆ ☆ ☆

WATER INTAKE (GLASSES)

⬭ ⬭ ⬭ ⬭
⬭ ⬭ ⬭ ⬭

"If it is important to you,
you will find a way. If
not, you'll find an excuse."
-Unknown

Intermittent Fasting Tracker

DAY		DATE		FASTING DAY	Y N	WEIGHT

FIRST BITE		FASTING HOURS	
LAST BITE		EATING HOURS	

SLEEP

TO BED		HOURS	
WOKE UP		SLEPT	

EXERCISE QUALITY

TIME		TYPE		DURATION	

MEAL / SNACK	TIME	CALORIES
	TOTAL	

ENERGY LEVEL

☆☆☆☆☆
☆☆☆☆☆

WATER INTAKE (GLASSES)

⬡⬡⬡⬡
⬡⬡⬡⬡

NOTES

"It does not matter how slowly you go as long as you do not stop."
-Confucious

Intermittent Fasting Tracker

DAY		DATE		FASTING DAY	Y N	WEIGHT	

FIRST BITE		FASTING HOURS	
LAST BITE		EATING HOURS	

SLEEP

TO BED		HOURS	
WOKE UP		SLEPT	

EXERCISE | QUALITY

TIME		TYPE		DURATION	

MEAL / SNACK	TIME	CALORIES
	TOTAL	

ENERGY LEVEL	NOTES
☆☆☆☆☆	
☆☆☆☆☆	
WATER INTAKE (GLASSES)	
⬭⬭⬭⬭ ⬭⬭⬭⬭	

"If it is important to you,
you will find a way. If
not, you'll find an excuse."
-Unknown

Intermittent Fasting Tracker

DAY		DATE		FASTING DAY	Y N	WEIGHT	

FIRST BITE			FASTING HOURS	
LAST BITE			EATING HOURS	

SLEEP

TO BED		HOURS	
WOKE UP		SLEPT	

EXERCISE QUALITY

TIME		TYPE		DURATION	

MEAL / SNACK	TIME	CALORIES
	TOTAL	

ENERGY LEVEL	NOTES
☆☆☆☆☆	
☆☆☆☆☆	

WATER INTAKE (GLASSES)

⬭ ⬭ ⬭ ⬭
⬭ ⬭ ⬭ ⬭

"It does not matter how slowly you go as long as you do not stop."
-Confucious

Intermittent Fasting Tracker

DAY		DATE		FASTING DAY	Y N	WEIGHT	

FIRST BITE		FASTING HOURS	
LAST BITE		EATING HOURS	

SLEEP			
TO BED		HOURS	
WOKE UP		SLEPT	

EXERCISE		QUALITY	
TIME		TYPE	DURATION

MEAL / SNACK	TIME	CALORIES
	TOTAL	

ENERGY LEVEL	NOTES

ENERGY LEVEL

☆☆☆☆☆
☆☆☆☆☆

WATER INTAKE (GLASSES)

⬤ ⬤ ⬤ ⬤
⬤ ⬤ ⬤ ⬤

NOTES

"If it is important to you, you will find a way. If not, you'll find an excuse."
-Unknown

Intermittent Fasting Tracker

DAY		DATE		FASTING DAY	Y N	WEIGHT	

FIRST BITE		FASTING HOURS	
LAST BITE		EATING HOURS	

SLEEP

TO BED		HOURS	
WOKE UP		SLEPT	

EXERCISE   QUALITY

TIME		TYPE		DURATION	

MEAL / SNACK	TIME	CALORIES
	TOTAL	

ENERGY LEVEL

☆☆☆☆☆
☆☆☆☆☆

WATER INTAKE (GLASSES)

⬠⬠⬠⬠
⬠⬠⬠⬠

NOTES

"It does not matter how slowly you go as long as you do not stop."
-Confucious

Intermittent Fasting Tracker

DAY		DATE		FASTING DAY	Y N	WEIGHT	

FIRST BITE		FASTING HOURS	
LAST BITE		EATING HOURS	

SLEEP

TO BED		HOURS	
WOKE UP		SLEPT	

EXERCISE

		QUALITY	
TIME		TYPE		DURATION	

MEAL / SNACK	TIME	CALORIES
	TOTAL	

ENERGY LEVEL	NOTES
☆☆☆☆☆	
☆☆☆☆☆	

WATER INTAKE (GLASSES)

⬤ ⬤ ⬤ ⬤
⬤ ⬤ ⬤ ⬤

*"If it is important to you,
you will find a way. If
not, you'll find an excuse."*
-Unknown

Intermittent Fasting Tracker

| DAY | | DATE | | FASTING DAY | Y | N | WEIGHT | |

| FIRST BITE | | | FASTING HOURS | |
| LAST BITE | | | EATING HOURS | |

SLEEP

| TO BED | | HOURS | |
| WOKE UP | | SLEPT | |

EXERCISE QUALITY

| TIME | | TYPE | | DURATION | |

MEAL / SNACK	TIME	CALORIES
	TOTAL	

ENERGY LEVEL	NOTES
☆☆☆☆☆ ☆☆☆☆☆	

WATER INTAKE (GLASSES)

⬡⬡⬡⬡
⬡⬡⬡⬡

"It does not matter how slowly you go as long as you do not stop."
-Confucious

Intermittent Fasting Tracker

DAY		DATE		FASTING DAY	Y N	WEIGHT	

FIRST BITE		FASTING HOURS	
LAST BITE		EATING HOURS	

SLEEP			
TO BED		HOURS	
WOKE UP		SLEPT	

EXERCISE		QUALITY	
TIME		TYPE		DURATION	

MEAL / SNACK	TIME	CALORIES
	TOTAL	

ENERGY LEVEL	NOTES
☆☆☆☆☆ ☆☆☆☆☆	
WATER INTAKE (GLASSES)	
⬭⬭⬭⬭ ⬭⬭⬭⬭	

"If it is important to you,
you will find a way. If
not, you'll find an excuse."
-Unknown

Intermittent Fasting Tracker

DAY		DATE		FASTING DAY	Y N	WEIGHT	

FIRST BITE		FASTING HOURS	
LAST BITE		EATING HOURS	

SLEEP

TO BED		HOURS	
WOKE UP		SLEPT	

EXERCISE		QUALITY	
TIME		TYPE	DURATION

MEAL / SNACK	TIME	CALORIES
	TOTAL	

ENERGY LEVEL

☆☆☆☆☆
☆☆☆☆☆

WATER INTAKE (GLASSES)

◊ ◊ ◊ ◊
◊ ◊ ◊ ◊

NOTES

"It does not matter how slowly you go as long as you do not stop."
-Confucious

Intermittent Fasting Tracker

DAY		DATE		FASTING DAY	Y N	WEIGHT	

FIRST BITE		FASTING HOURS	
LAST BITE		EATING HOURS	

SLEEP			
TO BED		HOURS	
WOKE UP		SLEPT	

EXERCISE		QUALITY	
TIME		TYPE		DURATION	

MEAL / SNACK	TIME	CALORIES
	TOTAL	

ENERGY LEVEL	NOTES
☆ ☆ ☆ ☆ ☆	
☆ ☆ ☆ ☆ ☆	

WATER INTAKE (GLASSES)

◊ ◊ ◊ ◊
◊ ◊ ◊ ◊

"If it is important to you, you will find a way. If not, you'll find an excuse."
-Unknown

Intermittent Fasting Tracker

DAY		DATE		FASTING DAY	Y N	WEIGHT	
FIRST BITE			FASTING HOURS				
LAST BITE			EATING HOURS				

SLEEP				
TO BED		HOURS		
WOKE UP		SLEPT		

EXERCISE		QUALITY		
TIME		TYPE		DURATION

MEAL / SNACK	TIME	CALORIES
	TOTAL	

ENERGY LEVEL	NOTES
☆☆☆☆☆ ☆☆☆☆☆	

WATER INTAKE (GLASSES)

◇◇◇◇
◇◇◇◇

"It does not matter how slowly you go as long as you do not stop."
-Confucious

Intermittent Fasting Tracker

DAY		DATE		FASTING DAY	Y N	WEIGHT	

FIRST BITE		FASTING HOURS	
LAST BITE		EATING HOURS	

SLEEP			
TO BED		HOURS	
WOKE UP		SLEPT	

EXERCISE		QUALITY	
TIME		TYPE	DURATION

MEAL / SNACK	TIME	CALORIES
	TOTAL	

ENERGY LEVEL	NOTES
☆☆☆☆☆ ☆☆☆☆☆	
WATER INTAKE (GLASSES) ◊◊◊◊ ◊◊◊◊	

"If it is important to you, you will find a way. If not, you'll find an excuse."
-Unknown

Intermittent Fasting Tracker

DAY		DATE		FASTING DAY	Y N	WEIGHT	
FIRST BITE			FASTING HOURS				
LAST BITE			EATING HOURS				

SLEEP				
TO BED		HOURS		
WOKE UP		SLEPT		

EXERCISE		QUALITY		
TIME		TYPE		DURATION

MEAL / SNACK	TIME	CALORIES
	TOTAL	

ENERGY LEVEL

☆☆☆☆☆
☆☆☆☆☆

NOTES

WATER INTAKE (GLASSES)

⬭⬭⬭⬭
⬭⬭⬭⬭

"It does not matter how slowly you go as long as you do not stop."
-Confucious

Intermittent Fasting Tracker

DAY		DATE		FASTING DAY	Y N	WEIGHT	

FIRST BITE		FASTING HOURS	
LAST BITE		EATING HOURS	

SLEEP

TO BED		HOURS	
WOKE UP		SLEPT	

EXERCISE | | **QUALITY**

TIME		TYPE		DURATION	

MEAL / SNACK	TIME	CALORIES
	TOTAL	

ENERGY LEVEL	NOTES
☆☆☆☆☆ ☆☆☆☆☆	

WATER INTAKE (GLASSES)

◊ ◊ ◊ ◊
◊ ◊ ◊ ◊

"If it is important to you, you will find a way. If not, you'll find an excuse."
-Unknown

Intermittent Fasting Tracker

DAY		DATE		FASTING DAY	Y N	WEIGHT	

FIRST BITE			FASTING HOURS	
LAST BITE			EATING HOURS	

SLEEP

TO BED		HOURS	
WOKE UP		SLEPT	

EXERCISE QUALITY

TIME		TYPE		DURATION	

MEAL / SNACK	TIME	CALORIES
	TOTAL	

ENERGY LEVEL

☆☆☆☆☆
☆☆☆☆☆

WATER INTAKE (GLASSES)

◯◯◯◯
◯◯◯◯

NOTES

"It does not matter how slowly you go as long as you do not stop."
-Confucious

Intermittent Fasting Tracker

DAY		DATE		FASTING DAY	Y N	WEIGHT	

FIRST BITE			FASTING HOURS	
LAST BITE			EATING HOURS	

SLEEP

TO BED			HOURS	
WOKE UP			SLEPT	

EXERCISE QUALITY

TIME		TYPE		DURATION	

MEAL / SNACK	TIME	CALORIES
	TOTAL	

ENERGY LEVEL	NOTES
☆☆☆☆☆ ☆☆☆☆☆	

WATER INTAKE (GLASSES)

⬠⬠⬠⬠
⬠⬠⬠⬠

"If it is important to you, you will find a way. If not, you'll find an excuse."
-Unknown

Intermittent Fasting Tracker

| DAY | | DATE | | FASTING DAY | Y N | WEIGHT | |

| FIRST BITE | | FASTING HOURS | |
| LAST BITE | | EATING HOURS | |

SLEEP

| TO BED | | HOURS | |
| WOKE UP | | SLEPT | |

EXERCISE QUALITY

| TIME | | TYPE | | DURATION | |

MEAL / SNACK	TIME	CALORIES
		TOTAL

ENERGY LEVEL	NOTES

☆☆☆☆☆
☆☆☆☆☆

WATER INTAKE (GLASSES)

◊ ◊ ◊ ◊
◊ ◊ ◊ ◊

"It does not matter how slowly you go as long as you do not stop."
-Confucious

Intermittent Fasting Tracker

DAY		DATE		FASTING DAY	Y N	WEIGHT	

FIRST BITE		FASTING HOURS	
LAST BITE		EATING HOURS	

SLEEP

TO BED		HOURS	
WOKE UP		SLEPT	

EXERCISE QUALITY

TIME		TYPE		DURATION	

MEAL / SNACK	TIME	CALORIES
		TOTAL

ENERGY LEVEL	NOTES
☆☆☆☆☆ ☆☆☆☆☆	

WATER INTAKE (GLASSES)

◯◯◯◯
◯◯◯◯

*"If it is important to you.
you will find a way. If
not. you'll find an excuse."
-Unknown*

Intermittent Fasting Tracker

DAY		DATE		FASTING DAY	Y N	WEIGHT	

FIRST BITE			FASTING HOURS	
LAST BITE			EATING HOURS	

SLEEP				
TO BED			HOURS	
WOKE UP			SLEPT	

EXERCISE			QUALITY		
TIME		TYPE		DURATION	

MEAL / SNACK	TIME	CALORIES
	TOTAL	

ENERGY LEVEL

☆☆☆☆☆
☆☆☆☆☆

NOTES

WATER INTAKE (GLASSES)

◊ ◊ ◊ ◊
◊ ◊ ◊ ◊

"It does not matter how slowly you go as long as you do not stop."
-Confucious

Intermittent Fasting Tracker

DAY		DATE		FASTING DAY	Y N	WEIGHT	

FIRST BITE		FASTING HOURS	
LAST BITE		EATING HOURS	

SLEEP

TO BED		HOURS	
WOKE UP		SLEPT	

EXERCISE QUALITY

TIME		TYPE		DURATION	

MEAL / SNACK	TIME	CALORIES
		TOTAL

ENERGY LEVEL

☆☆☆☆☆
☆☆☆☆☆

WATER INTAKE (GLASSES)

⬤⬤⬤⬤
⬤⬤⬤⬤

NOTES

"If it is important to you, you will find a way. If not, you'll find an excuse."
-Unknown

Intermittent Fasting Tracker

DAY		DATE		FASTING DAY	Y N	WEIGHT	

FIRST BITE			FASTING HOURS	
LAST BITE			EATING HOURS	

SLEEP				
TO BED		HOURS	
WOKE UP		SLEPT	

EXERCISE		QUALITY		
TIME		TYPE		DURATION

MEAL / SNACK	TIME	CALORIES
	TOTAL	

ENERGY LEVEL	NOTES
☆☆☆☆☆ ☆☆☆☆☆	

WATER INTAKE (GLASSES)

◊ ◊ ◊ ◊
◊ ◊ ◊ ◊

"It does not matter how slowly you go as long as you do not stop."
-Confucious

Intermittent Fasting Tracker

DAY		DATE		FASTING DAY	Y N	WEIGHT	

FIRST BITE		FASTING HOURS	
LAST BITE		EATING HOURS	

SLEEP

TO BED		HOURS	
WOKE UP		SLEPT	

EXERCISE QUALITY

TIME		TYPE		DURATION	

MEAL / SNACK	TIME	CALORIES
		TOTAL

ENERGY LEVEL

☆☆☆☆☆
☆☆☆☆☆

WATER INTAKE (GLASSES)

◊◊◊◊
◊◊◊◊

NOTES

"If it is important to you, you will find a way. If not, you'll find an excuse."
-Unknown

Intermittent Fasting Tracker

DAY		DATE		FASTING DAY	Y N	WEIGHT	

FIRST BITE			FASTING HOURS	
LAST BITE			EATING HOURS	

SLEEP				
TO BED			HOURS	
WOKE UP			SLEPT	

EXERCISE		QUALITY		
TIME		TYPE		DURATION

MEAL / SNACK	TIME	CALORIES
	TOTAL	

ENERGY LEVEL

☆☆☆☆☆
☆☆☆☆☆

WATER INTAKE (GLASSES)

○○○○
○○○○

NOTES

"It does not matter how slowly you go as long as you do not stop."
-Confucious

Intermittent Fasting Tracker

DAY		DATE		FASTING DAY	Y N	WEIGHT	

FIRST BITE		FASTING HOURS	
LAST BITE		EATING HOURS	

SLEEP

TO BED		HOURS	
WOKE UP		SLEPT	

EXERCISE QUALITY

TIME		TYPE		DURATION	

MEAL / SNACK	TIME	CALORIES
		TOTAL

ENERGY LEVEL

☆☆☆☆☆
☆☆☆☆☆

WATER INTAKE (GLASSES)

◯◯◯◯
◯◯◯◯

NOTES

*"If it is important to you,
you will find a way. If
not, you'll find an excuse."*
-Unknown

Intermittent Fasting Tracker

DAY		DATE		FASTING DAY	Y	N	WEIGHT	

FIRST BITE		FASTING HOURS	
LAST BITE		EATING HOURS	

SLEEP

TO BED		HOURS	
WOKE UP		SLEPT	

EXERCISE QUALITY

TIME		TYPE		DURATION	

MEAL / SNACK	TIME	CALORIES
	TOTAL	

ENERGY LEVEL

☆☆☆☆☆
☆☆☆☆☆

WATER INTAKE (GLASSES)

◯◯◯◯
◯◯◯◯

NOTES

"It does not matter how slowly you go as long as you do not stop."
-Confucious

Intermittent Fasting Tracker

DAY		DATE		FASTING DAY	Y N	WEIGHT	

FIRST BITE		FASTING HOURS	
LAST BITE		EATING HOURS	

SLEEP

TO BED		HOURS	
WOKE UP		SLEPT	

EXERCISE		QUALITY	
TIME		TYPE		DURATION	

MEAL / SNACK	TIME	CALORIES
		TOTAL

ENERGY LEVEL

☆☆☆☆☆
☆☆☆☆☆

WATER INTAKE (GLASSES)

◯◯◯◯
◯◯◯◯

NOTES

"If it is important to you, you will find a way. If not, you'll find an excuse."
-Unknown

Intermittent Fasting Tracker

DAY		DATE		FASTING DAY	Y N	WEIGHT	
FIRST BITE				FASTING HOURS			
LAST BITE				EATING HOURS			

SLEEP					
TO BED			HOURS		
WOKE UP			SLEPT		

EXERCISE			QUALITY		
TIME		TYPE		DURATION	

MEAL / SNACK	TIME	CALORIES
	TOTAL	

ENERGY LEVEL	NOTES
☆☆☆☆☆ ☆☆☆☆☆	

WATER INTAKE (GLASSES)

◇ ◇ ◇ ◇
◇ ◇ ◇ ◇

"It does not matter how slowly you go as long as you do not stop."
-Confucious

Intermittent Fasting Tracker

DAY		DATE		FASTING DAY	Y N	WEIGHT	

FIRST BITE		FASTING HOURS	
LAST BITE		EATING HOURS	

SLEEP

TO BED		HOURS	
WOKE UP		SLEPT	

EXERCISE QUALITY

TIME		TYPE		DURATION	

MEAL / SNACK	TIME	CALORIES
	TOTAL	

ENERGY LEVEL	NOTES
☆☆☆☆☆	
☆☆☆☆☆	

WATER INTAKE (GLASSES)

◊ ◊ ◊ ◊
◊ ◊ ◊ ◊

"If it is important to you, you will find a way. If not, you'll find an excuse."
-Unknown

Intermittent Fasting Tracker

DAY		DATE		FASTING DAY	Y N	WEIGHT	
FIRST BITE			FASTING HOURS				
LAST BITE			EATING HOURS				

SLEEP				
TO BED		HOURS		
WOKE UP		SLEPT		

EXERCISE		QUALITY			
TIME		TYPE		DURATION	

MEAL / SNACK	TIME	CALORIES
	TOTAL	

ENERGY LEVEL

☆☆☆☆☆
☆☆☆☆☆

WATER INTAKE (GLASSES)

⬤ ⬤ ⬤ ⬤
⬤ ⬤ ⬤ ⬤

NOTES

"It does not matter how slowly you go as long as you do not stop."
-Confucious

Intermittent Fasting Tracker

DAY		DATE		FASTING DAY	Y N	WEIGHT	

FIRST BITE		FASTING HOURS	
LAST BITE		EATING HOURS	

SLEEP			
TO BED		HOURS	
WOKE UP		SLEPT	

EXERCISE		QUALITY	
TIME		TYPE	DURATION

MEAL / SNACK	TIME	CALORIES
		TOTAL

ENERGY LEVEL	NOTES
☆☆☆☆☆	
☆☆☆☆☆	
WATER INTAKE (GLASSES)	
⬡⬡⬡⬡ ⬡⬡⬡⬡	

"If it is important to you,
you will find a way. If
not, you'll find an excuse."
-Unknown

Intermittent Fasting Tracker

DAY		DATE		FASTING DAY	Y N	WEIGHT	

FIRST BITE		FASTING HOURS	
LAST BITE		EATING HOURS	

SLEEP			
TO BED		HOURS	
WOKE UP		SLEPT	

EXERCISE		QUALITY	
TIME		TYPE	DURATION

MEAL / SNACK	TIME	CALORIES
	TOTAL	

ENERGY LEVEL

☆☆☆☆☆
☆☆☆☆☆

WATER INTAKE (GLASSES)

⬭⬭⬭⬭
⬭⬭⬭⬭

NOTES

"It does not matter how slowly you go as long as you do not stop."
-Confucious

Intermittent Fasting Tracker

DAY		DATE		FASTING DAY	Y N	WEIGHT	

FIRST BITE		FASTING HOURS	
LAST BITE		EATING HOURS	

SLEEP			
TO BED		HOURS	
WOKE UP		SLEPT	

EXERCISE		QUALITY	
TIME		TYPE		DURATION	

MEAL / SNACK	TIME	CALORIES
	TOTAL	

ENERGY LEVEL	NOTES
☆☆☆☆☆	
☆☆☆☆☆	
WATER INTAKE (GLASSES)	
⬤⬤⬤⬤ ⬤⬤⬤⬤	

"If it is important to you, you will find a way. If not, you'll find an excuse."
-Unknown

Intermittent Fasting Tracker

DAY		DATE		FASTING DAY	Y	N	WEIGHT	

FIRST BITE		FASTING HOURS	
LAST BITE		EATING HOURS	

SLEEP			
TO BED		HOURS	
WOKE UP		SLEPT	

EXERCISE		QUALITY		
TIME		TYPE		DURATION

MEAL / SNACK	TIME	CALORIES
	TOTAL	

ENERGY LEVEL

☆☆☆☆☆
☆☆☆☆☆

WATER INTAKE (GLASSES)

◊ ◊ ◊ ◊
◊ ◊ ◊ ◊

NOTES

"It does not matter how slowly you go as long as you do not stop."
-Confucious

Intermittent Fasting Tracker

DAY		DATE		FASTING DAY	Y N	WEIGHT	
FIRST BITE				FASTING HOURS			
LAST BITE				EATING HOURS			

SLEEP			
TO BED		HOURS	
WOKE UP		SLEPT	

EXERCISE			QUALITY	
TIME		TYPE		DURATION

MEAL / SNACK	TIME	CALORIES
		TOTAL

ENERGY LEVEL

☆☆☆☆☆
☆☆☆☆☆

WATER INTAKE (GLASSES)

◊ ◊ ◊ ◊
◊ ◊ ◊ ◊

NOTES

"If it is important to you, you will find a way. If not, you'll find an excuse."
-Unknown

Intermittent Fasting Tracker

DAY		DATE		FASTING DAY	Y N	WEIGHT	

FIRST BITE			FASTING HOURS	
LAST BITE			EATING HOURS	

SLEEP

TO BED		HOURS	
WOKE UP		SLEPT	

EXERCISE QUALITY

TIME		TYPE		DURATION	

MEAL / SNACK	TIME	CALORIES
	TOTAL	

ENERGY LEVEL

☆☆☆☆☆
☆☆☆☆☆

WATER INTAKE (GLASSES)

◇ ◇ ◇ ◇
◇ ◇ ◇ ◇

NOTES

"It does not matter how slowly you go as long as you do not stop."
-Confucious

Intermittent Fasting Tracker

DAY		DATE		FASTING DAY	Y N	WEIGHT	
FIRST BITE				FASTING HOURS			
LAST BITE				EATING HOURS			

SLEEP				
TO BED			HOURS	
WOKE UP			SLEPT	

EXERCISE			QUALITY	
TIME		TYPE		DURATION

MEAL / SNACK	TIME	CALORIES
	TOTAL	

ENERGY LEVEL	NOTES
☆☆☆☆☆ ☆☆☆☆☆	

WATER INTAKE (GLASSES)

◇ ◇ ◇ ◇
◇ ◇ ◇ ◇

"If it is important to you, you will find a way. If not, you'll find an excuse."
-Unknown

Intermittent Fasting Tracker

DAY		DATE		FASTING DAY	Y N	WEIGHT	

FIRST BITE		FASTING HOURS	
LAST BITE		EATING HOURS	

SLEEP

TO BED		HOURS	
WOKE UP		SLEPT	

EXERCISE QUALITY

TIME		TYPE		DURATION	

MEAL / SNACK	TIME	CALORIES
	TOTAL	

ENERGY LEVEL

☆☆☆☆☆
☆☆☆☆☆

WATER INTAKE (GLASSES)

◊◊◊◊
◊◊◊◊

NOTES

"It does not matter how slowly you go as long as you do not stop."
-Confucious

Intermittent Fasting Tracker

DAY		DATE		FASTING DAY	Y N	WEIGHT	

FIRST BITE		FASTING HOURS	
LAST BITE		EATING HOURS	

SLEEP			
TO BED		HOURS	
WOKE UP		SLEPT	

EXERCISE		QUALITY	
TIME		TYPE		DURATION	

MEAL / SNACK	TIME	CALORIES
	TOTAL	

ENERGY LEVEL	NOTES
☆☆☆☆☆	
☆☆☆☆☆	

WATER INTAKE (GLASSES)

◊ ◊ ◊ ◊
◊ ◊ ◊ ◊

"If it is important to you, you will find a way. If not, you'll find an excuse."
-Unknown

Intermittent Fasting Tracker

DAY		DATE		FASTING DAY	Y N	WEIGHT	

FIRST BITE		FASTING HOURS	
LAST BITE		EATING HOURS	

SLEEP

TO BED		HOURS	
WOKE UP		SLEPT	

EXERCISE QUALITY

TIME		TYPE		DURATION	

MEAL / SNACK	TIME	CALORIES
	TOTAL	

ENERGY LEVEL

☆☆☆☆☆
☆☆☆☆☆

WATER INTAKE (GLASSES)

◇ ◇ ◇ ◇
◇ ◇ ◇ ◇

NOTES

"It does not matter how slowly you go as long as you do not stop."
-Confucious

Thank You

Thank you for your purchase! If you enjoyed this book, please consider dropping us a review. It takes 5 seconds and helps small businesses like ours.

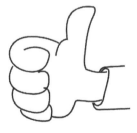

Made in United States
Troutdale, OR
02/20/2024